Personal Stories of Diet and Weight Loss and How They Do and Don't Work

with Foreword by Tommy L. Howell

For people who believe "it's their season" to lose weight.
For my husband and his tremendous support in writing this book.
For Bradley S. Nelson and "the intervention" that changed my life.

This book expertly edited by Tammie L. Retherford.

Foreword

About eight years ago, Harry and I went to Cedar Point amusement park which advertises itself as the roller coaster capital of the world. At the time, I weighed about 300 pounds. My experiences on roller coasters at Disney and Six Flags parks did not prepare me for the disappointment at Cedar Point and later Universal Studios. Out of 15 or so roller coasters I wanted to ride, I was only able to ride seven. From trying out the seat and safety mechanisms, I was able to determine that I could have ridden one more roller coaster for every ten pounds of weight I would need to shed. If I had lost eighty pounds, I expect I could have ridden every coaster without a problem.

When you are losing weight, one way to motivate yourself is to make plans for all the things you want to do in your newly trim body. I want to return to Cedar Point once I have lost those eighty pounds so that I can do all the things I missed out on before.

I have known Harry for over twenty years. In that time, we have both struggled with our weight. Sometimes we have dieted together and other times we each tried something the other was unwilling to try, but were always supportive of each other's efforts. I'm pleased to tell you that I personally know many of the contributors to this book and have also celebrated their successes and consoled them in whatever way they failed. Some of their stories are heartbreaking with related health problems that interfere with their ability to lose weight and some are unexpectedly hopeful after decades of being morbidly obese. I want you to know that whatever your struggle with your weight, you are not alone. Having a support system of friends and family makes a huge difference in your ability to make permanent changes to your situation.

Read these stories with an open mind and an open heart. Be sensitive to other people about their weight. Be supportive without nagging or guilt. If you need to lose weight yourself, my last advice is to maintain a positive "can do" attitude, especially in the face of setbacks.

Tommy Howell

Author of "Level Up Your Cooking: 12 Fresh Herbs to Boost Flavor and Health"

Introduction

      This is a very unique book not because the subject is about diet and weight loss—there are THOUSANDS of books out there on these topics—but because of the stories of the people who have experienced them. This is a book about those who decided to do something about their weight, and their experiences following the diets, weight loss, or weight management programs they had chosen. This book contains no sales pitches from diet, weight loss, or weight management creators, doctors, nurses, health professionals, chefs, or nutritionists—only first-hand accounts from people who have succeeded (and failed). They offer their advice. After reading these stories, we'll look at the similarities of the experiences observed and attempt to draw some conclusions about what approaches you might consider if and when you decide to lose weight, too.

      You may have noticed that I use the terms *diet* and *weight loss / weight management* separately as if they are different topics. This is because they are different approaches to losing weight. The Merriam-Webster dictionary defines a *diet* as "a regimen of eating and drinking sparingly so as to reduce one's weight" and is typically delivered in the form of a book. There is seemingly no formal definition for *weight loss* or *management program*, but what makes these "a program" are the addition of external influencing mechanisms, such as exercising, maintaining a food diary, having access to a blog or chat room, going to meetings, listening to audio and video training sessions, and drawing support from others following the same program. In addition to these differences, *successful* weight loss and weight management programs rely on a *change in eating and life habits* and usually cost considerably more than a diet book.

So which approach to losing weight works best? Is it an inexpensive book or an expensive program? After all, don't you get what you pay for? If that's true, then if you pay a small amount of money for a diet book, should you expect to get small and short term results? Conversely, if you spend hundreds on a weight loss or management program, isn't it logical to expect large and lasting results? Based on my own personal struggle and the struggles of the contributors in this book who have lost and gained weight, they followed these methods. We say no to this rationale. As for me and my contributors, we deal with the selection and conformation of diets and weight loss and management programs in "living color" not in black and white terms.

So to add food for thought as it were, consider some of the other factors involved in the selection and conformation of a diet, weight loss, or weight management program. To make this simple and straight forward, here are some of the more common questions people consider when preparing to make the decision to lose weight.

1. Which program should I try first (or next)?
2. How long will I need to stick to a program in order to reach my weight loss goal?
3. Once I've lost the excess weight, how will I keep it off?
4. How much will-power and self-discipline will it take for me to follow the program?
5. What foods will I have to give up on the program?
6. What foods will I have to learn to like on the program?
7. Will I need to remove "forbidden foods" from my kitchen?
8. Will I still be able to drink alcohol and lose weight?
9. Will I have to exercise on the program, and assuming so, for how long and how often?
10. Do I have to see my doctor before I start the program (especially for those with health conditions like high blood pressure, high cholesterol, arthritis, or others)?
11. Can I count on my family and friends to support or sabotage my efforts?
12. How do I handle eating out, especially at buffets?
13. How do I follow the program during holidays and observances to keep from gaining weight?
14. How do I follow the program while on vacation or a business trip?

15. As I do lose weight, should I put away or give away my "big" clothes in favor of smaller sizes?

Of course this list doesn't cover all the possible questions people ask before going on a diet or weight loss / management program, but I think you get the idea. The cost is not the only consideration people make when selecting a program. Many of these and other questions were asked of the people contributing their personal stories in this book. Many of their stories cover multiple diets and attempts at losing weight, with some achieving their weight loss goal while some are still working on it.

Dieters succeed and fail on diets and weight loss / management programs for a variety of reasons. Some people succeed because of their determination, medical or other necessity, desire to look and feel better, and/or need for self-fulfillment. On the other hand, people fail at losing weight for an equal number of reasons including medical issues, lack of determination, self-conceived lack of necessity, contentment with their appearance, or not being able to address the answer to any number of the above questions.

But there's one specific reason why people don't succeed at losing weight—one of the most important—it's just not their *season*, that is to say, they just aren't ready emotionally. Now don't confuse not being ready emotionally to lose weight with a lack of will-power or self-discipline. Naturally losing weight is a slow process, and as such, a person needs to reach a place in his or her life, or *be in his or her season*, when he or she says, "I must to lose weight for...whatever reason(s)." To demonstrate what I mean, let me start by sharing my own personal account of my struggles to lose weight.

My Story

Here are the basics: I am a married, white male between 45-54 years old. I've spent about $400 for the weight management program I'm following now, and I've given away about $100 in "big" clothes and food since I've been following the program. Since the start I've lost 65 pounds in six months. I've had to rely on some self-discipline and will power, have reduced intake of sugary foods and haven't had to eat foods I don't like. I have had to remove some sugary foods from my kitchen to keep the temptation of eating them at bay, and I don't drink much alcohol on the program but never have anyway.

I exercise regularly and eat out often. Since my husband and I follow the plan together, and we have no children, it's easy to support each other. We know ourselves enough to realize that we aren't likely to follow strictly the program during holidays or on vacation.

Growing up, I never had a weight problem, even though I ate what I wanted, when I wanted, and how much I wanted. My parents were heavy, but since I was adopted, maybe that contributed to me being a normal-sized child. I did ride my bike and walk a lot since I didn't get a car until I was 20 years old. Throughout my 20s, I still remained a normal weight for my size, but also I remained active with lots of walking since school and employment kept me busy.

In my 30s, I started taking jobs that were more sedentary in nature, so I slowly began to gain weight. I first noticed the weight around my belly, but later, other areas began to increase in size. Also, I met my current husband and found that we both enjoyed similar foods and snacks. We spent a lot of time together doing sedentary activities, so my weight slowly continued to increase through my 40s and into my early 50s.

During these 20-plus years together, we tried several diets, usually twice each, in case we did it wrong the first time! Both of our weight decreased then increased each time we went on and off various programs. We followed the Atkins Diet three times. During the first attempt, we lost about 30 pounds and then less on the other two tries, but each time we went off the diet the pounds came back on. We also tried the South Beach and Liver Cleansing diets twice, and lost some weight, but when we got off of them, we gained it all back and then some.

About a year ago, I weighted in the 240s when I went to see my doctor. He asked me if I was going to try to lose weight, and based on my negative experiences with diets, I said I would only try if it was needed because of a life-threatening condition. The doctor said "well at least you're honest about it" and promptly put me on high blood pressure and cholesterol medications. I stayed on these prescriptions for about six months, and then went back for a check-up. I tipped the scales at 252 pounds and moved to XXL in shirt size and 44" waist pants, so I started buying "big" clothes.

I decided that if I was ever going to look and to feel good again, live a longer life, have a quality of life, and get off those darn medications that I HAD to lose weight, and thankfully it was my season to lose weight, so I tried a high protein shake program which was similar to Slim Fast. Although I was hungry a lot, I did manage to lose about ten pounds in two months. It was late August of 2015 when I heard about the weight management program I'm on as of the writing of this book. The new program was introduced to me in a rather unique way – through an intervention of sorts.

My future husband wanted a bachelor party with his friends, so I made arrangements to be "kidnapped" by my best friends, Brad and Denise, for an evening of food and games, then a sleep-over with my fiancé joining us for brunch the next day. Brad picked me up after work and took me to their home, and it was then that I was introduced to the program he had been following for a couple of months. Little did I know that my fiancé asked Brad if he would talk to me about the program since my future husband already had decided to give it a try. I knew Brad had been losing weight, so he was living proof that the program worked as do most of them. Usually the problem comes when you get off the diet because you revert back to the ways you ate before.

The program relies on sound principles to retrain the participant to lose weight, not by changing what they eat, but changing when and how they eat. You follow advice handed down for decades, which is to chew your food slowly and only eat when you are actually hungry. This new way of eating, combined with regular, moderate exercise has reduced my weight from 242 to 182 pounds in just eight months. My doctor said my target weight should be 170 pounds, so I still have 12 pounds to lose, but by following the program principles, I know I can reach my goal. Then once I do, I'll move into maintenance mode, which is nothing more than continuing to follow the program, but a few principles can be relaxed, so I'll stop losing weight and just maintain it.

When I went in for a checkup earlier this year, my doctor was amazed at my progress and asked what I was doing. He had never heard of the program, which I find strange since it's been around since the 1970s and has been peer reviewed by medical professionals and journals with very positive results. Interestingly enough, the program didn't even make the top 38 diets for 2016 according to U.S. News and World Report Best Diet Rankings!

I plan to continue following my new eating and walking habits for the rest of my life. I plan on doing it by eating what I want (except a lot less sugar). I plan on doing it slowly and eating only when I'm actually hungry. I am happier with myself than I've been in many years, and I love not having to eat diet foods, but instead, I eat what everyone else eats. The program is the best-kept weight management program on the Planet—but it shouldn't be!

• • • • • •

So what have we learned just by reading my story? Besides the basic demographical information, we've learned that I've spent several hundred dollars to participate in the program I'm on, and I've lost a significant amount of weight, admittedly partly based on reliance of will power and self-discipline, but I find it easier to do so because I feel it's *my season* to lose weight. I haven't had to change up much of the foods I eat, except sugary foods although I eat out often. I engage in moderate, regular exercise and have a support mechanism since my husband and like-minded friends encourage me to stay on the program. I'm happy and satisfied with the program, but realize that I could (and do) "fall off the wagon" at times, especially when on vacation and during holidays and observances.

So there's nothing really earth-shattering here, right? You're probably glad for my success and may go so far as to wish me well with my future weight loss goals. But how different is my experience from yours, my reader? There may be few or many differences, but to be fair, I'm a typical person. I never weighted over 300 pounds, nor have I so far been unable to lose excess weight. I don't have diabetes, a malfunctioning thyroid, or heart disease. So there's nothing really remarkable about my story. But as the old saying goes, "but wait...there's more"!

What follows are some stories that you may find remarkable and hopefully inspiring. But in the end, *AND IF IT'S YOUR SEASON*, you too may decide that it's time to follow a diet or weight loss or management program, and if you do, perhaps these stories will help you make an informed decision about which one to try—or to try next.

The ONE truth that I always want you to remember and never forget is this formula for losing weight:

WEIGHT LOSS = CALORIES IN < CALORIES BURNED

Realizing that not all calories are created equal, in simplest terms, you must take into your body less calories than those you burn in a given day, which is **about 2,000 for the average adult.** No matter which diet or weight loss or management program you decide to choose, the big picture is this formula and always has been the key to weight loss in whatever form it takes.

Now let me introduce you to some other people who have struggled with their weight and let me show you how their interesting and diverse stories may help you as you consider a diet or weight loss or management program for yourself.

Tamarah's Story

First, I'd like to introduce Tamarah. She is a married woman of American Indian/Alaskan Native heritage and is between 45 and 54 years old. The diet and weight loss programs she has been on include the Atkins Diet, Jenny Craig, the Medifast Diet, Nutrisystems, Slim-Fast, Weight Watchers, the Zone, Slim for Life, and one of her own creation. With nine diets tried and failed, I think it's safe to say that she's tried them all, as it were, so she has a good perspective on dieting. According to Tamarah, the "only one I lost weight on was my own diet, which was a starvation type diet. I lost 80 pounds in two months [and] I have never been able to replicate that weight loss."

The program she has tried most recently is the Maker's Diet, on which she lost four pounds in five days, but she is no longer on that one either because it "was too difficult to maintain [and] was exceedingly restrictive." The Maker's Diet regimen includes water in the morning, fruit, seeds, and nuts at noon; water and fruit at three o-clock, water and raw vegetables with no dressing at six o-clock, and water. "Nothing else at all. No salt, no sugar, no soda, no fun!" However, starting the diet didn't cost her any money because she went to a public library and checked out a book about it. She also didn't spend any money on giving away inappropriate food items or ill-fitting clothes simply because she couldn't maintain the program. She also had to eat raw vegetables, which wasn't a preferred way of taking in nutrition. She wasn't able to dine out either because all foods had to be in an all-natural state. Finally, Tamarah did not actively exercise while on the program.

After gathering the above basic information about her diet and weight loss experience, I asked her, as well as all of the contributors in this book, to tell me her story about her life-long struggle with weight loss and gain and the results she observed. What follows is Tamarah's account, in her own words.

I was born in 1968. Although I don't recall much prior to 1974, I do have latent issues related to food and my appearance, which first surfaced as early as two years of age. This was due to, in part, my mother's poverty and weight issue. Against my grandparents' advice and boisterous admonitions, my mother dropped out of high school and married a foreign-born man, who considered women as unworthy chattel. During her marriage from 1965-1970, my mother was physically abused and deprived of basic needs, such as food, running water, and electricity. This abuse eventually pervaded our home and everyone living there. I vaguely recall fighting the dogs for their dog food and eating kibble. In 1969, my grandparents took custody of me and my infant brother because we had no food and were starving. My grandmother later told me that I weighed about twelve pounds and my infant brother weighed about 6 and a half pounds, which was a pound and one-half less than his birth weight. One year later, my mother left her husband and moved back to her parents' (my grandparents) home. When we lived with our grandparents, we had plenty of good and nutritious food. My grandmother cooked all of our food. We regained our health, and we felt safe. In 1973, my mother met and married the man who adopted me and my brother and who I would know as my only father. Upon leaving the safety of my grandparents' home, my brother and I longed to return to their home.

Instead, we remained with our mother and adopted father. Soon, they had three more children of their own. During this time, my mother gained several hundred pounds and suffered many nervous breakdowns. By 1975, my mother weighed 450 pounds. I began to associate weight gain with mental disease. To compound problems, my mother did not work, nor did she take care of the home. She and my adopted father fought constantly. We had only starchy, unappetizing food that we drowned in jalapenos, mustard, or ketchup. The only fruit we had were mushy and bruised apples and tart, seedy oranges. In an effort to save money and food, my father put a locked bicycle chain on the door of the refrigerator, which infuriated our mother much more. In 1976, my mother asked me if I wanted to move out of the house with her, and I replied no. I wanted to either live with my grandmother or my adopted father. It was then that my mother told me that my adopted father was not my father. She went on telling me

16

that the only reason my father adopted me was because he was ashamed of me. She said that he did not think I was pretty; that my little sisters were much prettier because they were his children. At that moment, I consciously loathed my appearance and longed to look more like my father's children. It was also at this time that I became hypersensitive to my weight and to the foods that I consumed.

During the 1970s and 1980s, it was high fashion to be bone thin. Popular models, like Twiggy, Tiegs, and Imam, were all the rage. As a young child and pre-adolescent, I envied extremely thin people because they appeared happy and well-liked. Whereas, my mother, who was morbidly obese, was a miserable, unloving person, who many people did not like. As early as eight years of age, I wanted to wear a size 0. I wanted to be able to put my hands around my thighs. I wanted a twenty-three inch waist. From that point on and throughout the remainder of my childhood, one of the greatest fears I entertained was the fear of being fat even though I was a healthy, slim, and athletic girl.

As a teenager, I never achieved a size 0, but I was never larger than a size 6. When I see pictures of myself as a teen, I can't believe that I even thought I was unattractive or fat, but I did. I was a beautiful young woman with no self-esteem who felt unloved with the exception of my grandparents. It was also during this time that I had two distinct relationships with food: love and hate. When I was at my grandparents' home, I loved the food they prepared for us. The food at their home was fresh, colorful, healthy, balanced, and delicious. Food tasted so good; it was *wonderful. During our weekly visits, my grandmother taught me how to cook wonderful meals. I was seven years old when I made my first family meal at my grandparents' home. My grandparents were proud, and my siblings and my extended family fawned over my cooking, which made me feel special. Even to this day, my greatest point of pride resides in my ability to cook fantastic food that makes people around happy and satisfied. Despite the love of nutritious cuisine that my grandparents instilled in me, I hated my mother's cooking. Her cooking stood in stark contrast to my grandmother's cooking, which I never really understood since my grandmother taught her to cook as well. My mother hated cooking for her large family. She prepared the most unappetizing grey-smothered food one can imagine. Her meals were primarily comprised of ground beef, mushroom soup, canned peas, canned corn, and egg noodles in one bubbling pot of mess. This was our nightly meal. Furthermore, I hated all the meals we consumed at home with the exception of special occasions, such as birthday parties and holidays. Breakfast was always the same: Cheerios and skim milk. Lunch was always the same: bologna sandwich and a withered apple or a hardened orange. There was no diversity in our eating, and there was no restaurant-going at all. As we grew older, my mother developed more severe mental problems, and her ability to feed her family was almost eliminated. From the time I was 13 years old until I left home at age 17, the responsibility to cook dinner fell upon me. During this period, my family appreciated my* ability to make good food with such limited resources, but my mother expressed jealously and hostility toward me. Her verbal and emotional abuse finally drove me out of the house at age 17.

When I turned 17, I got married to my high school sweetheart who went into the US Navy. For the second time in my life, I felt safe and well cared for. We had plenty of food, and I cooked food for my husband. I was still thin, weighing only 120 pounds at the time. I gave birth to my first child when I was 18 years old. I gained only 65 pounds with her, and I quickly lost the weight. Unfortunately, when my daughter was one year old and I was pregnant with my second child, I had a car accident that killed my daughter and my youngest sister. The baby I was carrying survived, but he was born with major disabilities—he would later pass away. After the car accident, I gained over 80 pounds because I had a broken back and was restricted to the bed. I depended on others to bring me food. I was very depressed and personally devastated. When I was released from the hospital, I discovered that my husband was unfaithful, and we divorced. I saw myself in the mirror, weighing almost 200 pounds. The thing I feared the most; I had become—fat.

It was at this time that I embarked on my weight loss escapade that would last for the rest of my life. The first diet I ever devised was my own starvation diet, which I would not recommend—ever! I did, however, lose all of the weight, but I deprived myself of everything. I only ate salad and one baked potato a day. Needless to say, I lost 80 pounds in 8 weeks. Slowly, I recovered mentally and physically. I gained some self-confidence, finally. I began my education. I met the man that I would eventually marry. I had three more children, and I remained at a healthy weight—never getting above 130 pounds after the end of my pregnancies. This amazed me because I ate whatever I wanted to eat. After losing the weight, I stayed at or below 130 pounds. At the time, I thought that I had conquered my weight problem, but I was VERY wrong.

After the birth of my fifth child, I went down to 125 pounds—like usual. When my last child was three months old, I noticed that my clothes were becoming tighter and tighter, day by day. That was odd, I thought. I began to monitor my weight, and I continued to gain a pound a day for about 120 days. Needless to say, I was alarmed—VERY alarmed. I went to the doctor. The doctor told me to stop eating food. I had not changed anything. I was very active. I walked every day. I ate reasonably. I cooked my food. What was the problem? The doctor checked my thyroid, which was on the low-normal side, but it was normal nonetheless. Within six months, I went from 125 pounds to 245 pounds, going from a size 7 to a size 18 in six months. I became exceedingly depressed. All of the negative feelings I had associated with obesity confounded my thinking. I became obsessed with dieting, willing to spend thousands of dollars if needed to be thin. Despite my crusade to eradicate this weight gain, my husband and children were very supportive, and they expressed their love for me even though I had gained weight. They still valued me; they still loved me even though I did not love myself.

For seventeen years, I have spent thousands of dollars trying to drop below 200 pounds. I went on Nutrisystem; I lost 40 pounds. I gained it all back when I stopped purchasing the food. I went on Jenny Craig; I did not lose any weight. I went on Medifast; I lost 40 pounds. I gained it all back when I went back to a full-food menu. I went on Adkins; I lost 40 pounds. I gained it all back when I began eating items that contained sugar. I went on the Zone diet; I lost no weight. I went on Slim for Life; I lost 20 pounds. I regained it after I stopped adhering to the diet plan. I joined Weight Watchers; I lost 20 pounds. I regained it after I stopped counting points. One time, I dropped 50 pounds, and I weighed less than 190 pounds. I did that when I stopped eating food for over a month. All I ate were two no-carb yogurts, one piece of broiled chicken, and a cup of steamed vegetables. I gained it all back when I began eating normally. I tried The Maker's Diet; I lost 5 pounds in four days. However, I could not maintain the restrictive diet. My highest weight was 252 pounds. Today, I weigh 230 pounds, but I eat what I want and when I want. I know that I am obese. If I lose the weight, then that will be great. If I don't, then I have accepted it. I no longer fear being overweight because I have learned that my value does not reside in my appearance. I have realized that my value comes from within my heart in how I treat and serve others. Perhaps one day, I will shed the weight that I am carrying since I understand how I have developed unhealthy perceptions about food and about my *appearance. Since I have stopped dieting, I have not weighed more than 230 pounds. Twenty-two pounds less than my highest weight is a start, and hopefully not a finish.*

As you have read, there can be many contributing factors to weight gain than just overeating and lack of exercise. In Tamarah's story, she had a number of outside influences contributing to her weight gain and loss. Her experience is a prime example of the proverbial yo-yo effect dieters suffer as they struggle to lose weight and keep it off. As of the writing of this book, she still struggles with her weight, and as yet, has not found a program that works for her.

Crystal's Story

This is Crystal, a single Asian woman between 35-44 years old. She has been on a number of diets and weight loss programs, including the Atkins Diet, the Blood Type Diet, the South Beach Diet, the Flat Belly Diet, Glycemic-Index Diet, Jenny Craig, Mediterranean Diet, Raw Food Diet, the Vegan Diet, Vegetarian Diet, and Weight Watchers. To date, none of these programs have worked for Crystal, again for various reasons. But in an effort to not give up on her health and wellness, she is now trying the Ayurvedic Diet and has as of the writing of this book lost six pounds. This diet simply provides a list of foods that you can eat; some frequently, some moderately, and some rarely.

She spent $20 to purchase the program book and hasn't yet given away any inappropriate foods or ill-fitting clothes. On this program Crystal has had to stop enjoying olive oil, olives, peppers and fruit, but she hasn't had to start eating things she doesn't typically like. She dines out about three times a month at casual and fine dining restaurants and selects only healthy options. Concerning exercise, Crystal says, "I do a lot of hiking for about an hour [each time]. When in the mountains, [I hike] every day. But when at home, I go for 40 minute walks to the store and back, twice a week."

What follows is Crystal's story, told in her own words, about her life-long struggle with weight gain and loss, including the problems she encountered while trying the TWELVE diet programs mentioned earlier.

When I was young, I was of average size for a kid. My mom never let us have sugary cereals or sweet snacks, and I was a bit of a tomboy always out playing football with the boys. My parents got us kids a trampoline and said it was the best gift they ever got us.

During my teens, I played lots of sports in school, but like most teenagers, I ate all kinds of junk food. However, I never had weight problems because I was so active.

Then I got married and had a baby when I was 20. I had pre-eclampsia during my pregnancy, which is a condition during pregnancy that causes a lot of stress on the baby and many health problems for the mom. One of the main things it does is causes too much weight gain very rapidly, and it causes water retention. After having my son, I had to have water drained from my body—over 40 pounds of water!

After having the baby, I worked out every day at the gym and started playing sports to help me get back my pre-baby body. I had gotten up to 204 pounds, but no matter how much I was exercising, I was not losing weight. My ex-husband was not very supportive and was constantly putting me down during pregnancy and afterwards. I was starving myself and losing my self-confidence and self-esteem. Finally, he ran off with another woman and left me broken in every way possible. At 22, I had been married, divorced and had a baby to take care of. I thought no one would ever love me or want me again. I was so depressed I didn't eat, and I would go run for 10 miles a day just to deal with the depression and stress. After a year of this, I had lost about 50 pounds and I was wearing a size 10, and I had begun to regain my self-esteem.

I started back to school to get my degree in my mid-20s. Because I was working full time and taking 21 semester hours, my eating was mostly fast food. By the time I finished my degree, I had gained 30 pounds and was back up to 180.

During my 30s, I had a high stress job, so I started being more health conscious and even became a vegetarian. I did one hour of yoga every night and would go walking for an hour on my days off. But even though I was eating little and exercising, I was just maintaining my weight. I tried the Adkins diet, the Blood Type diet, South Beach diet, and Mediterranean diet. I also tried different detox programs, acupuncture, natural weight loss pills, and over the counter weight loss pills, but with no positive effects.

I am now in my 40s, and I'm starting to have menopausal symptoms. I talked to my doctor, but he said I still have a few more years before that. I still hike and walk a lot, but my physical issues are still with me; all the while thinking they are just age-related problems. But as I was speaking to my sister about all these issues, she told me she too had many of the same problems. She said her doctor told her that women who have pre-eclampsia as she and I have, usually also have thyroid problems. So I had some medical *tests run and found that I have hypothyroidism. Although I had been tested for this condition before, the results were negative (barely), so it was dismissed in spite of having all the symptoms. Now the medical threshold has changed, hence the recent diagnosis. I still weigh between 175 and 180 pounds, and my doctor just put me on a two-month treatment to see how I respond. All-in-all though, I was glad to learn the primary reason for my weight gain, knowing that my physical condition strongly contributed and knowing it wasn't just a lack of poor nutrition and exercise. I look forward to eventually getting back to the weight I should be.*

As you've read, weight gain and loss can also be contributed to physical problems outside of basic diet and exercise regimens. Crystal wasn't aware of this as it pertained to her own body until she spoke to a blood relative about her issues, and only then realized that heredity was playing a role in her struggle to maintain a healthy weight.

She didn't explain the two-month treatment her doctor has her on to lose weight, but I feel certain the program takes into account her hypothyroidism condition because as we all know, there is no pill that will healthfully eliminate excess weight.

So far, the stories you have read show that determination, and to some extent will power, found their places in the telling, but as I alluded to earlier, these qualities alone will not help a person lose weight. The program you follow must be *sustainable* for lasting results.

Brad's Story

Allow me to introduce Brad. He is a married, white man between the ages of 45 and 54, but to date, he has only tried two diet and weight management programs: the Medifast Diet and a weight management program called Naturally Slim, or NS to abbreviate. Even though Brad's first-hand experience with structured diet and weight loss programs is limited, he nonetheless has a remarkable story to tell. As of the writing of this book, Brad has lost 78 pounds on NS, and he reports that he has no intention of quitting the program. Like all dieters, he has a target weight in mind, and he's counting on the principles he learned in NS to help him achieve his goal.

Naturally Slim doesn't *require* it's participants to count calories, points or carbohydrates, but instead teaches the overeater a new way to eat the foods he or she enjoys most. In Brad's case, his employer paid for his participation in NS, so he's had no out-of-pocket expenses to participate, but he has donated between 100-200 dollars of food he no longer eats and ill-fitting clothes he can no longer wears due to his significant weight loss. The only foods he has given up on the program are soups and most sugary items; otherwise, he eats only the foods he enjoys. He dines out several times a week and eats the foods he likes at restaurants, as well. Exercising amounts to Brad doing elliptical training 30 minutes a day and walking 10,000 steps daily, or as close to it as he can, which he monitors with his Fitbit. With this introduction, here's Brad's story, in his own words.

I had been overweight since literally the third grade, if not before. As I progressed into (young) adulthood, it just got worse until I found myself at nearly 400 pounds when I was 24 years old. After speaking with a co-worker who had lost a good amount of weight, I started the Medifast plan which, at the time, meant drinking three sweet (chocolate, vanilla or strawberry) shakes per day, and no solid food whatsoever. I somehow managed to do this for almost 9 months and lost all the way down to 225 pounds. But then I got off of the diet, and the weight came back. By 1999, I had gained it all back, plus some, and was admitted into the hospital for a leg infection, weighing in at over 500 pounds!

After that, I managed to lose some on my own, and through another diet or two, but never really did anything notable to try to lose weight in an organized way. I had been diagnosed with type II diabetes and a number of other related conditions and was insulin dependent.

Finally, in June of 2015, I was looking through my wellness program at my office and saw Naturally Slim. It was free for me to take through them, and it gave me some wellness points (which, in turn, offered discounts on insurance premiums). I decided to try the program, starting at a weight of 299 pounds.

Much to my shock and disbelief, the weight started falling off in leaps and bounds, while still eating my favorite foods. Before I knew it, I had blown past my initial goal of 40 pounds lost, and had completely gotten off of insulin injections. As of March 2016, I'm down to 221 pounds and feeling fantastic. I literally have not weighed this little since I was in high school and maybe even before that.

My goal is to lose another 40-50 pounds to get myself into a "normal" BMI, but I'm not going to try to rush it. The beauty of Naturally Slim is that maintenance mode is almost identical to weight loss mode, so it's easier to make it a life-long thing. I never really did well on programs that forced me to give up certain foods (e.g. carbs, fats etc.), they're just not sustainable.

I have found my lifelong weight management program in Naturally Slim.

As Brad said, NS is *sustainable*, meaning that because "It's not WHAT you eat, but WHEN and HOW you eat that will help you lose weight", a person following NS doesn't have to change the foods he or she eats; just how much and how often. As Brad also pointed out, maintenance mode is just basically following the NS principles but relaxing a few of them, so you don't continue to lose weight once you have reached your target goal.

Because Naturally Slim is a program based solely on information, I am not legally authorized to reveal any of the core principles of the program in this book, and indeed, everything stated thus far has come from materials openly offered by NS and freely available to the general public through the NS web site and on social media services like YouTube.

Please don't think that the goal of this book is to sing the praises of Naturally Slim, but instead remember the title of the book, which discusses diet and weight loss programs and how they do and don't work—through personal accounts by people who have experienced them first-hand. I know NS will be discussed further by my contributors, but *so will other diet and weight loss programs*. Indeed, several other programs have been and will be mentioned multiple times, but as you read further, you may observe that NS seems to be the one program with little or no criticism and posits praises of success by those who follow it.

A word about my contributors. To obtain contributors for this book, advertisements were placed on Facebook and Reddit, along with blog entries on the TiVo Community Forum to recruit participants, so a wide audience was polled. It's interesting to note that many of those choosing to contribute to this book also happen to be on the NS program. I had trouble finding contributors who succeeded on other programs, which I think makes an important statement and ties directly into the focus of this book. My goal was to get a cross-section of dieters to participate as contributors, but instead, I kept finding people that only wanted to talk about their experiences on Naturally Slim.

Ilana's Story

This is Ilana's story. She's a Hispanic/Latino married woman between 35-44 years old. The programs she has tried include the Atkins Diet, Glycemic-Index Diet, Nutrisystems, the Paleo Diet, and Weight Watchers. She, too, is currently on Naturally Slim. According to Ilana, the "Weight Watchers' Core Plan worked well as did Nutrisystem's but as soon as I stopped, the weight came back. I lost about 30 pounds with each and then hit a wall. Naturally Slim has been a revelation. I have *easily* lost 53 pounds, and I am still losing. I have another 30 pounds or so to go, but I know I will lose it this year...and keep it off!"

Ilana spent about $400 for the NS program and has donated about $500 of inappropriate foods and ill-fitting clothes due to her significant weight loss. Her food choices really haven't changed since following NS, and she "eats out several times per week. Most [restaurants] are casual dining or fast food." Her exercise consists of routinely walking about 12,000 steps per day for her job." So let's find out why Ilana's story is significant when it comes to losing weight.

My name is Ilana S., and I am 38 years old. I am a married mother of two elementary school aged children. I have struggled with my weight since I was in middle school and reached puberty. I was bullied throughout high school because of my weight, and I feel that it has always defined who I am as a person and that my weight affected my definition of my self-worth.

In my early 20s, I was diagnosed with PCOS (Polycystic Ovary Syndrome) and a metabolic disorder. While the diagnosis helped me explain why I had an extraordinarily hard time losing weight, no doctor was able to give me a strategy to be able to lose weight successfully and keep it off. Some diets proved to be more successful than others. I joined Weight Watchers and used their Core plan so that I wouldn't have to count points or measure food. I lost about 30 pounds, but after getting pregnant with my first child, I never went back to it.

I had two children and three years of difficulties with gestational diabetes. Luckily, I was not diabetic when I was pregnant, but I always struggled with insulin resistance and pre-Diabetes. When my youngest child was two, I tried Nutrisystem. I hated the food but was able to again lose about thirty pounds. But with the expense of the program and the limited food options, I stopped after about six months.

Then, one year ago exactly, I had a wake-up call. I reached my highest weight of 225 pounds. At under 5'0" tall, this was a serious threat to my health. I also saw a picture of myself, and I couldn't understand who that fat person in the picture was. This isn't who I truly am. I cut back on my food and started walking...and between March and June of 2015, I lost about 12 pounds. Then, at the end of June, I was introduced to the *Naturally Slim* plan through an online forum I participate in. I joined immediately and at the end of the ten week program, I reached my goal of 20 pounds lost.

Now, I have lost a total of 53 pounds, and I am still losing. I started out wearing a size 18/20/2X. I just bought a dress and jeans in a size 10! Now I look at pictures of myself and don't recognize the thin person I see, and it is a wonderful feeling. Best of all, my husband was inspired by my success and joined NS. He has lost 46 pounds and is still losing. I know that we are setting healthy examples for our children, and we are now an active, healthy family. We go hiking, we travel, and our lifestyle has completely changed for the better.

Based on Ilana's story, I'd say she felt it was her *season* to lose weight when she hit 225 pounds. Have you noticed the triggers that get people to decide once and for all that they need to lose weight? Sometimes it's a medical reason, reaching certain number displayed on a bathroom scale, or sometimes it's a comment made that causes a person to say "I don't want to be known as that". For me, it was a combination of the number on the scale and comments made. I entered my *season* when I reached 252 pounds on the doctor's office scale, and I heard a second hand comment made from an employee of a restaurant I frequent. I typically go to a certain restaurant with a female friend, but one day she went with her family instead of me, and the greeter asked her, "Where's the *big guy*"? I didn't want to be known as "the big guy", and so entered *my season* to losing weight.

To reinforce the major points of this book requires us to remember that the primary issues with most programs mentioned so far is that, although they work to help a person lose weight, there are issues with some programs that prevent the person from *maintaining* a new weight, and as a result, regain the weight, and in some cases, with a vengeance. Again, diet and weight loss and management programs not only need to help you lose weight, but also they need to be *sustainable for a lifetime* to help you keep the weight off while promoting feelings of *happiness and satisfaction*.

Next up is Rex's story. It's short, and to the point, but nonetheless a meaningful part of recounting the experiences of people who struggle to lose excess weight and to keep it off.

Rex's Story

Rex is a partnered, white male between 55-64 years old who has previously followed the Ornish Diet but who also is on Naturally Slim. When I interviewed, Rex he told me that he lost 70 pounds following the Ornish low-fat diet along with an exercise program back in his 40s. Since being on NS, he's lost 20 pounds. As mentioned earlier, NS doesn't require a person to count calories, points, or carbohydrates, and according to Rex, "counting calories is a daunting task and almost impossible to keep up on a long term basis." This is a facet of dieting that many people dislike, perhaps because counting these kinds of measurements just makes life in general that much more cumbersome.

Alex's partner paid for the NS program, which he follows, as well. Alex said that as of yet, he has not donated any of his smaller size jeans because "he wants to be sure the weight loss sticks this time."

The inappropriate food Alex has chosen to give up include: "cookies and sweets, diet soda, processed foods, and anything with trans fats." Some of these were given up by choice, not by NS mandate, because the mantra of the program is, "It's not WHAT you eat, but WHEN and HOW you eat that will help you lose weight." Giving up cookies and sweets along with trans fats is recommended, but diet sodas and processed foods are allowed. In fact, all foods are allowed on NS, but in smaller portions and with less frequency. Also, Alex admits that he dines out 3-5 times a week, and when eating out, he avoids fast food restaurants and tries to eat at dine-in restaurants.

Alex's exercise regimen includes walking 4-5 times per week on the treadmill or around the neighborhood. He says, "I go to the gym two or more times per week for upper and lower body weight training. For variety, I mix up my walking with the elliptical, bicycle riding, tennis, indoor rowing and swimming. My fitness tracker and [heart rate] monitor have become critical items in my fitness quest." Fitness trackers like Fitbit and Jawbone have been increasing in popularity over the past year and are great tools to help a person stay motivated. I recently purchased one of these to help me track how many steps I take each day. I strive for 10,000 steps a day, and since I don't want to count that high on and off all day long, I let my monitor do it for me. These activity trackers also act as accountability measures and encourages you to meet your daily exercise goals.

With all of the above comments in mind, and in a brief but to-the-point recitation, here is Rex's personal account of his weight management activities.

I was never overweight until my late twenties when my eating habits caught up with me, and I started to gain weight. Being a self-help book junkie, I began to exercise and learn more about the foods and exercise I needed to keep healthy.

Unfortunately, I have become the epitome of a yo-yo dieter. I have lost up to 70 pounds on three occasions, only to put the weight (and often more) back on once I stopped exercise and watching my food intake.

I have never really followed a diet program specifically [until now]. Through my reading, I know what I should and should not be eating and the exercise I need to do to stay fit. I am currently using the Naturally Slim program to support the efforts of my partner and to see if the key principles of the program can help me make a lifestyle change that sticks this time.

I'm sure Rex can and will lose the weight he desires to lose, while maintaining good health and vitality, if he will continue to follow the NS core principles as a permanent part of his lifestyle, because that's how NS was designed to work—as a *sustainable,* lifelong way of eating and living.

Eddy's Story

      Eddy is a Hispanic/Latino, married man between 45-54 years old. To date the programs he's tried include: the Atkins Diet, the Paleo Diet, the South Beach Diet, and the Whole30 Diet. He, like a number of the others interviewed, is currently on Naturally Slim, on which Eddy "has lost 50 pounds so far (after already having lost 30 on the 'starve yourself as much as you can bear' diet plan)." He spent $400 to enroll in NS and because of his significant weight loss, has had to replace all of his clothes. He dines out "once or twice a week, and goes out for pizza, sushi, and Mexican cuisine, which are among his favorites." Eddy walks for an hour with his dogs 4-5 days a week, with no other exercise. Now in his own words, here's Eddy's story.

      I am a married, 54 year old white Hispanic male. I've spent about $400 for the weight management program I'm following now, and I've given away pretty much all of my wardrobe since I've been following the plan. I have lost about 50 pounds (and counting), and this after having worked very hard with a more traditional diet to lose 30 pounds before I started on this plan. While the plan does not restrict any specific foods, it has trained me to reduce my sugar intake and to eliminate snacking altogether.

38

I exercise regularly but lightly, walking my dogs for an hour most, but not all, days. My wife is also on the same plan, so it makes it easier. I sometimes travel and try to keep to the general principles when I do, but it is sometimes hard.

Growing up, I was not obese, but I was always on the chubby side. I was always the "fat" brother. I did some sports, and I pretty much did not worry about my weight. When I got to college, I was still in that range and stayed there since I did a lot of walking, intramural sports and kept reasonably active (and had no money to eat out!). I was probably around 200 pounds and wore 34" waist pants.

I got married right after graduation and started work as a software engineer, which meant sitting at a computer all day. My wife is a good cook, so I started to gain weight. There was no huge or fast increase, just steadily, a few pounds a year. After 25 years, I crept up to my top weight of about 265 pounds. I was wearing 42-44" waist pants; I had high blood pressure, high cholesterol, back issues (those started as a teen, and got worse as my weight increased), and my health, while not terrible, was not great.

I needed to lose some weight, and my brother, a doctor, was really pushing me, and offered a nice TV if I could bring my weight under 200 pounds. So for a year, I went on a "starvation" diet. Since I am a very picky eater, none of the traditional diets would really work for me (too many foods I would not tolerate). So I cut down my intake severely, and counted every calorie that touched my mouth. And the pounds came off. In a year, I reached 199.8, and claimed my prize. That was nine years ago. There was only one problem, and that was that I hated my life every day of that diet. I was hungry and miserable. I could not eat many of the foods I liked. Eating was a chore, and not a pleasure. So the next day, I went "off" the diet, thinking to myself that maybe I could just add a few things I liked and I would not be so miserable. In two years, I was back at my old weight of 263 pounds!

Six years passed while I played a yo-yo with my weight, losing and regaining the same 20-30 pounds, over and over. My doctor kept on telling me I needed to get to about 220 pounds for my health, but I never could get there.

In January of 2015, I had some lab tests that scared the heck out of me. My cholesterol was high (even with meds). My triglycerides were sky high, my liver numbers were not great, and my "pre-diabetic" A1C numbers had crept into the "go on medication" levels. I swore to my doctor that I would lose some weight and make it stick. So I went back on starvation mode, and after a few months was down to 230. I knew I could not sustain the loss regime, so I went on "maintenance" mode. At least I was not gaining, but I was not happy either and not eating the foods I really wanted.

This continued for six months, and I figured this was as good as it would get. But during those months, I had been hearing about this Naturally Slim plan that a lot of my friends were on. And they were losing weight. Some were losing amazing amounts of weight. And all of them kept on saying how easy it was; how they could eat any foods they wanted, and how they would be able to do this plan for the rest of their lives. It sounded ridiculous. It sounded like magic. It sounded like a cult! But I was desperate.

So I went on NS in late September, and it changed everything. It taught me how to eat, so that I could eat all the things I loved, and still lose weight in a way that was sustainable. Six months in, I have lost over 50 pounds and now weight about 180. I'm wearing 32"waist pants. I was in high school the last time those numbers were that low! I do not feel deprived, and I feel like my eating habits have permanently changed. So I will never be "off the diet" since I do not feel I am on a diet in the first place. I just eat differently.

I went to the doctor last week for my checkup. He had not seen me for eight months. I have been seeing this same doctor 15 years, and he even lives next door to my brother, so he knows me outside the office. He walked by my room a couple of times on the way to see other patients, glanced in, but didn't say anything, which was very strange. But when he walked in, he explained he had not recognized me! To say he was astounded would be an understatement. My lab numbers were all in the normal range, and he said he took the hypertension and pre-diabetes diagnosis off my chart. He was practically giddy since he had watched me on the diet roller-coaster for so many years.

With just a few more pounds lost, I will be in the normal BMI (body mass index) range for my height and weight; something which I thought was never achievable for decades. I sometimes look at myself in the mirror and don't recognize the reflection. I eat all the foods I love. I go out to *dinner without fear of overeating. I have desserts when I want them. And I feel great. I can truly say that NS changed my life.*

Now I need to go buy more clothes; I just had to donate another bunch that I outgrew, or under-grew, as the case may be.

Eddy, too, determined that it was his *season* to lose weight after getting such poor blood test results after his medical exam. His was a real life wake-up call, with the realization that if he didn't change the way he ate, his quality of life would continue to decrease, right along with his health. I had a similar experience with my last doctor visit as Eddy did, but the difference with mine was that I was far more excited about the significant weight I had lost than my doctor was after badgering me for years to lose weight! It was just another day in the life of a general practitioner for him, I guess, but it was a celebration for me!

Sue's Story

Sue is a married, white woman between 45 and 54 years old. The programs she has tried include: Jenny Craig, the Richard Simmons Deal-a-Meal audio/video program, and Seattle Sutton (similar to Nutrasystem), and she tried a food sensitivity plan created just for her by her doctor and nutritionist. According to Sue, "Jenny Craig made me ill, but I lost about 50 pounds in four months." When she stopped the program, she gained the weight back within the next six months. Furthermore, she says that "the food sensitivity plan allowed me to lose 75 pounds in eight months, and I'm much healthier overall because of it", but she is no longer following that plan either.

She now follows the Oxford Biomedical Technologies LEAP Plan for those with food sensitivity concerns. So far, she has lost 77 pounds. This plan requires Sue to log everything she eats, but there are no calories or grams to count. For this program, she has spent $295; plus, she has paid for three nutritionist visits at $180 each, for a total of $835. She has lost enough weight that she has had to do a number of alterations to keep from buying smaller clothes. She has had to give up almost all of the foods she enjoys, and she has learned to eat buckwheat, cumin, beets, and lima beans. She rarely dines out and does not maintain a regular exercise regime due to health issues. With the preliminaries out of the way, here's Sue's story.

Here are the basics: I am a married, white female between 45-54 years old. I've spent about $295 for the weight loss program I'm following now and about $600 on visits to the nutritionist. I've had to take in a bunch of clothes (thankfully I can sew!) since I've been following the LEAP plan. Since starting LEAP, I've lost over 75 pounds.

Growing up I always had a weight problem. My parents were heavy, and I never learned how to eat healthy.

In my 20s, I'd gain and lose weight like a yo-yo doing things like excessive exercise and only eating broiled chicken and vegetables but never following a specific plan.

In my early thirties, I met my now husband and found that we had a mutual love of food. I was diagnosed with a disease called Pseudo Tumor Cerebi and was advised to lose weight - PRONTO! I spent several hundred dollars to become a lifetime member of Jenny Craig. Over the course of a few months, I became increasingly ill but utilized Jenny Craig foods. I lost about 60 pounds in about six months. My disease did not resolve with the weight loss, and I ended up having major surgery to assist with the illness. After the wedding and honeymoon, I realized I actually felt better eating non-Jenny Craig food, so I decided to discontinue the plan.

Over the next decade, the weight crept back on. I'd push a bit to get my pants to button again, but the weight kept coming back. I was working full time, juggling health issues and eating what and how much I wanted. Hubby suggested we try Seattle Sutton just because he'd heard it was good food and easy. Over the course of a few months, I did lose weight, but I was having issues with headaches and stomach pains. After a long vacation, I felt better, so my doctor suggested I stop Seattle Sutton saying that maybe something in the process was bothering me.

In my early 40s, I had more issues with Pseudo Tumor Cerebi. I learned that the major surgery I had a decade before was failing. Once again, I had to have major surgery. During the next two years, I had 13 surgeries. I was suffering from chronic daily migraines and a never-ending headache. My weight ballooned, and doctor after doctor failed in helping me find relief.

Finally, my long time neurologist said "I don't know what to tell you next" and sent me to a functional medicine neurologist. She spent a lot of time explaining to me how functional medicine works and a lot of issues are usually based in your gut. I started a standard elimination diet from The Institute of Functional Medicine. It seemed pretty easy— I could eat as much as I wanted as long as it was an approved food. After several months of incorporating this process, I'd lost some weight but felt horrible. At this point, we discontinued the diet, and the doctor sent me to a nutritionist. I continued to eat mainly foods from the prior plan but also treated myself to meals out plus some extra goodies. Weirdly, I started to feel better.

The nutritionist suggested that we run some food sensitivity testing. My blood was drawn and sent to Oxford Biomedical Technologies. Based on my results (which SHOCKED me) I started a new elimination diet that allowed me to eat foods that wouldn't irritate my intestinal system. At this time, I'm continuing on the elimination diet, and in the seven months since I first saw the functional medicine neurologist, I've lost over 75 pounds. Although I weigh more than I did on my wedding day, my dress is too big (I'm waiting to alter it down, so I only have to do it once). I still have more to go, but I will continue downward. My current goal is to be in "OneDerLand", that is be below 200 pounds by 2017.

This is certainly one of those instances where a person MUST seek medical advice before starting a diet or exercise program. In fact, Sue had to consult with several medical professionals before finding a program that worked for her. It seems she is happy with her results and the LEAP program, and isn't that what really matters? Losing weight, exercising to stay fit, living a healthy lifestyle, avoiding sugar, and so on are all part of the journey to a healthy you. If the program you are on is *sensible* and *sustainable*, helps you lose the excess weight while promoting a feeling of *happiness and satisfaction*, and then has a built-in method of allowing you to *maintain* your new weight *for the rest of your life*, then that's the perfect formula for a viable diet or weight loss or management program. Don't look solely at cost, reputation, and popularity of a program, but rather look for *evidence* that the program works and is sustainable for a lifetime *from people who follow it.*

Sheryl's Story

My final story comes from Sheryl, a single, white female between 45-54 years old. The diets and weight loss programs she's followed include: the Paleo Diet, Weight Watchers, and the Whole30 Diet. According the Sheryl, "All three have been successful for me. [Weight Watchers] helped me lose and maintain a healthy weight for many, many years using the Points system. However, I was diagnosed with Type 2 diabetes about four years ago (a genetic issue triggered by my heart stopping), and even with the help of a nutritionist, I had trouble controlling carb intake. I tried Whole30 almost two years ago, and [I]lost about 20 pounds. I [continue] to follow the Paleo Diet, which has kept both my weight and [blood test] numbers low." She has lost 25 pounds on Paleo to date.

Sheryl also told me that on Paleo, there "is no measuring. Basically it's either yes or no. Either I can have [a food], or I can't." She didn't spend any money to buy program books or materials but has given away about $500 in ill-fitting clothes and inappropriate foods because of following the diet. Concerning food, she's had to give up "processed sugar, artificial sweeteners, dairy, and carbs like pasta, rice, potatoes, and bread. Fortunately, I like almost everything. I eat meat, fowl, fish, beans, eggs, nuts, vegetables, and fresh fruit. I like it all, but I miss carbs." As for dining out, Sheryl goes wherever she likes because she "can always find meat and veggies to eat".

For exercise, she goes to the gym four times a week. During three of her four visits, she "power [walks] on the treadmill for about 45 minutes. The fourth time is a class— either Spin or Body Sculpting (we alternate weeks)." Sheryl's story will be of special interest to those with heart disease and diabetes, and her success with her weight loss programs.

I am almost 55 years old (next month!), and I have been on a diet most of my life. Food has been my best friend, and my worst enemy. I was a skinny little kid, but I began gaining weight around age ten and never looked back. I was a fat adolescent, a fatter young adult, and an even fatter adult. I tried everything: the old Weight Watchers, Think Thin, Atkins, the Grapefruit Diet—you name it, I tried it. I even worked as a counselor at a weight loss camp. Everything worked—for a while. But eventually, everything failed, and I ended up higher on the scale than before.

When I turned 25, something clicked. I remember crying on my 25th birthday because I was so unhappy, and I just said ENOUGH. Over the next seven months, I dropped over 70 pounds— no specific program, but I was a professional dieter at that point, so I knew what I should and shouldn't be eating. I added in a pretty rigorous exercise program. I swam for an hour every morning, walked about six miles a day, and did toning exercises every morning (crunches, etc.). I looked great, and I felt great, and it lasted for about five years.

After that the weight would creep up and down—never as bad as before, but I see-sawed about 25-30 pounds on a regular basis. I finally found the Weight Watcher points system, and it worked great for me. I stayed on it for many years with great success. I knew I would always diet, and it was a good plan for life where I could eat well but still enjoy certain foods in moderation.

When I turned 50, I had a life altering event. My heart stopped in the middle of Manhattan's Penn Station. I was lucky enough to be in a crowded place where help was close, and I was miraculously revived with the help of extensive CPR and a portable defibrillator. As it turns out, I had a bunch of clogged arteries. The doctors were very surprised that someone my age, with my level of fitness (I was slim!) had this issue, but they discovered I had a genetic condition called familial hypercholesterolemia. Basically, no matter what I ate or how well I took care of myself, only medication could help. Well, that and a triple bypass. The surgery went well, but another genetic factor had kicked in due to the trauma— I also had a family history of diabetes, and the heart failure kicked it into gear. So I left the hospital with two new health conditions: heart disease and diabetes.

After several months of trying different medications, we finally got the cholesterol under control. The diabetes was another problem. At first, I seemed to have it under control as well, until my A1C [blood glucose number] jumped to a TEN and scared the crap out of me! I knew I had to do something drastic. A friend of mine had been eating a Paleo diet for years and had gently suggested on a few occasions that it might help my diabetes. I called her and told her I was ready. She gave me a bunch of literature from her nutritionist and told me to go on the Whole30 website. I have been following the program ever since. Within the first three months, my A1C number dropped down to 7, and I lost over 20 pounds. It has been close to two years now, and I am still eating Paleo. My weight is low, but because my diabetes is genetic, I will always need to watch my diet and take medication. I allow myself the occasional cheat (some wine usually!), but I try to stick as closely to the plan as possible.

As always, I wish I could eat like "normal" people, but that has never been the case for me, and never will be. I will always need to control my diet, whether it be for my appearance or my health.

What a remarkable story about diet and weight loss! The Paleo and Weight Watchers diets helped Sheryl lose a significant amount of weight, and she has been able to keep the weight off for several years. How much of these programs rely on self-discipline and will power is unknown, but from her account she seems to be happy with her successes...so far. Being a diabetic and having heart disease will require Sheryl to take medications and to maintain a medical relationship with her physician for the rest of her life, but she has succeeded in losing excess weight and keeping it off, and sustainably so.

Similarities and Summary

Now that you've read the personal accounts of eight contributors who have all had good and not so good experiences with various diets and weight loss programs, I'd like to try and put the facts and figures raised into perspective, but first let me tell you a little about the contributors I used for this book.

As I mentioned at the end of Brad's story, I placed advertisements asking people to respond to a short survey about their personal experience with diet and weight loss on Facebook, Reddit, and the TiVo Community Forum. These ads were targeted at audiences interested in diet and weight loss, of which I received 25 responses. Of those, 17 indicated they were male and 8 were female, with the age range of all respondents between 35-64 years old. The following table shows how many respondents followed one or more of the top 38 diets for 2016 as published by the U.S. News & World Report Best Diet Rankings.

Diet or Weight Loss Program	Frequency	Popularity
Atkins Diet	10	1
The Engine 2 Diet	1	7
Flat Belly Diet	1	7
Glycemic-Index Diet	3	5
HMR Program	1	7
Jenny Craig Diet	4	4
Medifast Diet	3	5
Mediterranean Diet	1	7
Nutrisystem Diet	2	6
Ornish Diet	1	7
Paleo Diet	4	4
Raw Food Diet	1	7
South Beach Diet	3	5
Slim-Fast Diet	5	3
Vegan Diet	1	7
Vegetarian Diet	1	7
Weight Watchers Diet	8	2
Whole30 Diet	3	5
Zone Diet	2	6

A quick look above reveals that the Atkins Diet is the most popular, followed by Weight Watchers then Slim Fast. The Naturally Slim weight management program discussed throughout this book didn't make the U.S. News 2016 list, which was followed by 11 respondents.

My original goal was to find 10-12 contributors who had unique stories about a variety of diets and weight loss programs they had followed. The survey revealed a diverse list of programs that the participants are following now, and the results they are experiencing. As I collected responses to my initial survey that was advertised as mentioned earlier, they were such that I had to settle for eight contributors, due to the overwhelming responses that revealed the majority of them following Naturally Slim program.

So despite my best intentions, the contributing results seem to make the focus of this book about Naturally Slim, which was not my goal. However, with that said, the majority of my contributors following NS make a statement in that this program is not only popular, but also that their experiences are consistent with a successful and *sustainable* weight management program that promotes *happiness and satisfaction*.

I emphasize the feelings of happiness and satisfaction because these are very important when it comes to staying with a diet or weight loss program for a long period of time. Based on the contributing results experienced, Naturally Slim not only helps the follower lose weight, but also achieves this through a lifestyle change by shifting into the "when" and "how" mentality of the weight loss process, instead of the "what". Let me explain what I mean.

Many diet and weight loss programs dictate what and how much foods are to be consumed on the plan. Many times these foods come in the form of what many consider to fall under the "healthy" category of foods, such as salads, vegetables, fruit, legumes, nuts, certain oils, and lean or low fat proteins like poultry, fish, diary and tofu. Over a long period of time, eating these kinds of foods, along with an appropriate amount of exercise, will cause a person to lose weight. But the questions seem to beg, "Are they happy doing this", and "Do they find satisfaction with the food they eat"?

I know for me, the diets I tried never made me happy and satisfied because of the food restrictions I had to adhere to *even though* I lost weight following these programs. For me, it wasn't just important for me to lose weight, but I needed to feel happy and satisfied with how I was doing it on a daily basis. It's these considerations that make Naturally Slim different from the rest of the diets and weight loss programs out there. NS changes the "when" and "how" you eat food not the "what". Following the NS core principles, you can actually eat pizza, pasta, fried foods, burgers, and other popular cuisines while you lose weight, be happy and stay satisfied while doing it—and no more "diet" food!

But we must not forget that, although NS is "the best thing since sliced bread" and "the best kept secret on the planet", it must be followed with the blessings of your medical professional because as we read in Crystal's, Sue's and Sheryl's stories, their medical conditions made a difference in how they lost weight. We know there's no magic pill we can take to lose weight. Perhaps someday this will change, but for now, we must simply take in fewer calories than we burn each day to lose weight in whatever form that takes.

References

Atkins Diet at http://www.atkins.com.
Ayurveda Diet at
https://www.theayurvedaexperience.com.
Blood Type Diet at http://www.dadamo.com.
Facebook at http://www.facebook.com.
Fitbit at http://www.fitbit.com.
Flat Belly Diet at
http://flatbellydiet.flatbellydiet.com/flatbellydiet/54010/index?cm_mmc=DirectLoad-_-21day-_-54010-_-218856&keycode=218856.
Glycemic-Index foods located at
http://www.glycemicindex.com/. Glycemic-Index
books can be found online with many booksellers.
Jawbone at https://jawbone.com/.
Jenny Craig Diet at http://www.jennycraig.com.
LEAP Plan by Oxford Biomedical
Technologies at http://nowleap.com/leap.
Maker's Diet at http://www.makers-diet.net/.
Medifast Diet at http://www.medifast1.com.
Mediterranean Diet at http://www.ifmed.org/.
Merriam-Webster Dictionary at
http://www.merriam-webster.com.

Naturally Slim at http://www.naturallyslim.com.
Nutrisystems Diet at
http://www.nutrisystem.com.
Ornish Diet at http://ornishspectrum.com/.
Paleo Diet at http://thepaleodiet.com/what-to-eat-on-the-paleo-diet/#.Vw6u-PkrLcc.
Personal quotes from Karen Petty, Ph.D., Marcia Upson, N.P., and Brad Nelson.
Raw Food Diet at
http://www.thebestofrawfood.com/. Raw foodism diet books can be found online with many booksellers.
Reddit at https://www.reddit.com/.
Richard Simmons Deal-a-Meal program. Not commercially available but can be purchased on Amazon at http://www.amazon.com.
Seattle Sutton at
https://www.seattlesutton.com.
Slim-Fast Diet at http://slimfast.com.
SlimGenics (a.k.a. Slim for Life) Diet at
https://www.slimgenics.com.
South Beach Diet at
http://www.southbeachdiet.com.
TiVo Community Forum at
http://www.tivocommunity.com/tivo-vb/.
U.S. News & World Report, L.P. Wellness section. U.S. News Best Diet Rankings. Accessed Jan. 15, 2016 at http://health.usnews.com/best-diet.
Vegan Diet at
http://www.health.com/health/gallery/0,,20773383,00.ht

ml. Vegan diet books can be found online with many booksellers.

Vegetarian Diet at http://oldwayspt.org/resources/heritage-pyramids/vegetarian-diet-pyramid. Vegetarian diet books can be found online with many booksellers.

Weight Watchers Diet at https://www.weightwatchers.com.

Whole30 Diet at http://whole30.com/whole30-program-rules/.

YouTube at http://www.youtube.com.

Zone Diet at http://www.zonediet.com.

Note: It is suggested that you use an up-to-date web browser to access the above web sites since many of them do not display or function correctly on older browsers.